Corporate Yoga

By Subodh Gupta

Corporate Yoga Trainer

First Edition February 2008

Copyright @2008 by Subodh Gupta

All rights reserved. No part of this publication may be reproduced, stored or transmitted in any form or by any means without the prior written permission of the Author.

ISBN 978-0-9556882-2-5

Published by
Subodh Gupta
+44(0)7966275913
Headquarter: London (UK)
Email: info@subodhgupta.com
www.subodhgupta.com

Publisher Note:

The reader should not regard the recommendation and Yoga exercise expressed and described in this book as substitute advice of a qualified medical practitioner. It is also advisable that reader may learn the Yoga exercise initially in presence of qualified yoga trainer.

Acknowledgements

I am grateful to my parents and all my teachers who taught me at various stages of my life & shared with me their wisdom.

I am also thankful to Models: Simona Spazzini, Zosia Lesiecka and Barbara Tomasik for taking their time out of their busy schedule to help me to complete my book.

Content

Introduction 7

Part 1

Understanding Yoga Postures 10
Yoga Exercises & their Importance 11
How many min Yoga I need every day 13
What should I practice if I have only 15 min 13
Notes for Yoga Practitioners 14

Part 2

Yoga exercises recommended for busy Corporate

1. Neck: Forward and Back bending 17
2. Neck: Chin over Shoulder 19
3. Neck: Ear to Shoulder 21
4. Shoulder rotation 24
5. Hand Clenching 27
6. Hands Stretching 28
7. Eye Exercise 30
8. Cat Stretch 37
9. Half Sun Salutation 39
10. Full Sun Salutation 44
11. Single Leg Raise 51
12. Single Leg lock Pose 53
13. Spinal Twist 55
14. Dolphin Exercise 57
15. Shoulder Stand 60

16. Bridge Pose   64
17. Cobra Pose   66
18. Child Pose   69
19. Simplified Side Stretch   72
20. Final Relaxation   75

Part 3:

Wellness Monitor   80
Yoga Practice Record   81

Introduction:

This book of corporate yoga has been written considering the need of people who work in corporate sector.

Normally when we hear about yoga the first thought comes to mind is some sort of acrobatic postures which seem to be impossible to perform.

However in actual practice yoga has nothing to do with complicated postures as yoga practice is not about competition but keeping healthy body and mind to achieve higher purpose in life.

During my visits to various corporate organizations to teach yoga exercises, I came across mainly four types of issues people face apart from stress: the lower back pain, neck pain, sprain in fingers & forearms and weak eye sights because of long hours of sitting on chair and working on computer and blackberry.

This book contains simple yoga exercises which will help in relieving pain from lower back, neck, fingers and forearms. It will also help in making eye muscles stronger, releasing stress and keeping the blood pressure normal.

If you find yourself getting tired easily or stressed, you can improve this situation by simple yoga exercises and you will be amazed to see how quickly you can improve your stamina and reduce your stress level.

Simplified yoga postures described in this book can be practiced by everybody, whether you are young or old, beginner or advance, your body is stiff or you have never done yoga before, etc.

This book has 3 parts. First part of the book contains straight to the point understanding about yoga, second part is about gentle and moderate yoga exercises which can be practice by everybody and third part is for you to record your practice.

In the end I would like to say that practicing Yoga should be pleasant and enjoyable. If you do it regularly, gently with breath awareness it will certainly bring good health to you.

May all being be healthy.

Subodh Gupta

"Yoga means Union"

Part 1

Understanding about Yoga posture

The most important issue in Yoga practice is not flexibility and ability to do acrobatic postures, but awareness of the body and breath. *I repeat awareness of the body and breath.*

No matter how physically difficult posture you are able to do but if it is without your focused attention and awareness of breath then it is a practice of a beginner, however even if you are doing physically seemingly easy posture with complete awareness it is an advanced stage practice of yoga system.

In this book for understanding purpose yoga word is used for yogic physical postures.

Yoga Practice and its Importance

Yoga practice consists of series of gentle and moderate exercises for various body joints which are practiced along with breath awareness.

These exercises help in releasing stiffness and trapped energy in gentle, effective and safe way. These exercises also make our muscles relaxed, supple, strong and joints get loosen up.

You can notice many people in their 60's start having various joints pain, lower back pain, neck pain, etc. The reasons could be our bad sitting postures, unhealthy life style, lack of physical movement, etc.

Muscles which are not used regularly become weak over a period of time and joints become stiff and free flow of energy in the body is obstructed which later on in old age create various kinds of pain in the body at different locations.

Let's understand with the help of an example:

Water which is flowing freely in the river under the sunlight tends to remain fresh, however stagnant water in any pond tends to get stale and germinate mosquitoes. Similarly if energy is flowing freely in our body, our body tends to remain healthy and if energy is obstructed for a long time, it creates pain and disease.

Regular practice will certainly lead you towards healthy body and mind.

How many minutes of Yoga exercises I should practice every day?

Ideally the best approach is if you can include yoga exercises as part of your daily life i.e. every day 1 hour session.

All the exercises from number 1 to 20 mentioned in content section can be completed within 1 hour session.

However, considering busy life schedule in corporate sector and frequent flying at odd hours, sometimes it is not possible to do yoga exercise regularly. In that case I would suggest one can do practice at least 35 to 45 minutes 4 days a week (please practice from exercise no 1 to 13 and then relaxation exercise no 20).

What yoga exercises should I practice if I have only 15 minutes?

It is always better to practice even little of yoga exercises every day rather than not doing it at all.

If your schedule permits you only 15 minutes in a day, I would recommend you may practice from exercise no 1 to 9 and then exercise no 20.

Please always remember to practice relaxation (exercise no 20) at the end of each yoga session.

Notes for Yoga Practitioners

Breathing through nose or mouth: Always breathe through the nose with the awareness (unless specified by mouth). *Remember a simple concept that by nature, mouth is for eating and nose is for breathing.* Please do not try to reverse the nature functions. As you breathe in, know that you are breathing in. As you breathe out, know that you are breathing out. This will greatly enhance your general health and well-being.

Nose performs not only the breathing function but it filters the air, moisturise the air, warms the air, it can smell, it secretes the mucus and performs many more functions, etc.

Now think for a moment if the mouth can perform all these functions…..

Yes you are thinking correctly, mouth cannot perform all these functions, so please do not breathe through mouth unless specified in some special exercises.

Place of practice: It is good to practice in a room which is well ventilated. Please do not practice under a fan or direct sunlight.

Sitting Posture for Yoga: Any comfortable sitting position is ok. The main point is the body needs to be relaxed and back straight. Do not slump and do not lean forward. It is good to sit on a folded blanket or a cloth which is made from natural fibre.

In case if you find it difficult to sit on the floor in a cross leg sitting position, some of the yoga postures described in this book can also be practiced while sitting on the chair.

Relaxation: Whenever you feel tired during the practice of yoga exercises, please lie down on the floor on your back for 2 - 3 minutes and try to relax.

Practice Time of yoga: The best time for yoga practice is early morning during sunrise or around sunset (Yoga exercises should only be done after at least 3 hours of eating the food. For example if you want to do yoga exercises at 6pm in the evening then please make sure that your lunch should have been eaten by 3pm).

Awareness during Yoga: It is very important that while practicing yoga exercises, you are aware of your breath and body movement.

Any yoga posture without awareness of breath is a practice of a beginner.

Frequency of Practice: In my view yoga exercises should be practice every day, however if not possible then at least 4 days a week.

Cautions: If you are suffering from any kind of neck related pain, injury, hernia pain or have gone through any recent operation, please consult your doctor first before beginning any of the yoga exercises.

Please also remember that some of the yoga exercises (from exercise no 9 to 20) mentioned in this book are strictly **not recommended if you are going through pregnancy.**

Part 2

Yoga Exercises

Exercise 1
Neck: Forward and back bending

Preparation: Sit in a cross-legged pose with hands resting on your knees with back straight (*You can also sit on the chair with your back straight if you find sitting on the floor with cross leg position inconvenient to you*).

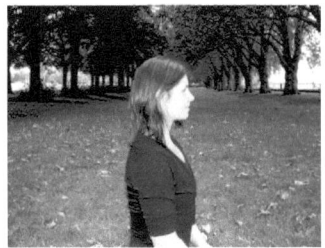

Caution: There should not be any strain in any neck movement. You can take your head forward and back only to the point where you feel absolutely comfortable.

Step1: As you exhale slowly bring your head down.

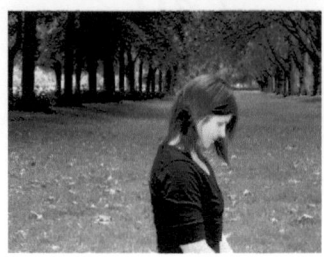

Step2: As you inhale move your head back as far as you feel comfortable.

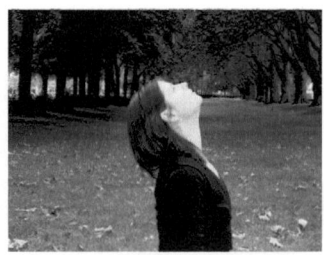

This is one round.

Practice 5 rounds.

Exercise2
Neck: Chin over shoulder

Preparation: Sit in a cross-legged pose with hands resting on your knees with back straight.

Step1: As you exhale turn your head towards your right shoulder.

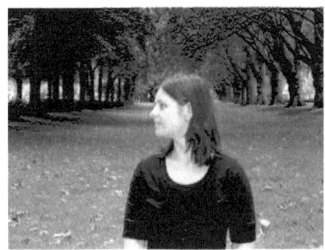

Step2: Inhale and bring the head to the centre position.

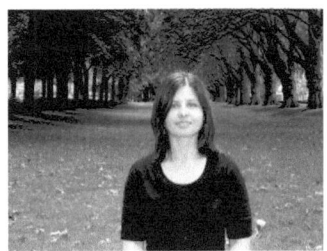

Step3: As you exhale turn your head towards your left shoulder.

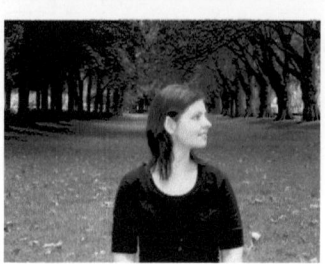

Step4: Inhale and bring the head to the centre.

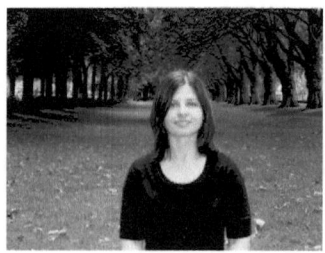

This is one round.

Practice 5 rounds.

Exercise 3
Neck: Ear to shoulder movement

Preparation: Sit in a cross-legged pose with hands resting on your knees with back straight.

Step1: As you exhale lower your head toward your right shoulder (lowering right ear towards your right shoulder as shown in the picture).

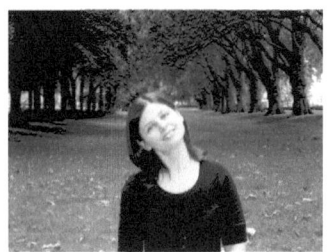

Step2: Inhale and come back to the centre.

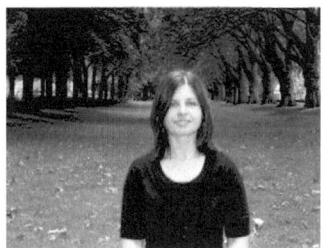

Model: Barbara Tomasik

Step3: As you exhale lower your head toward your left shoulder.

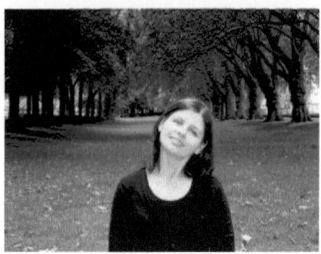

Step4: Inhale and come back to the centre (these 4 steps complete one round).

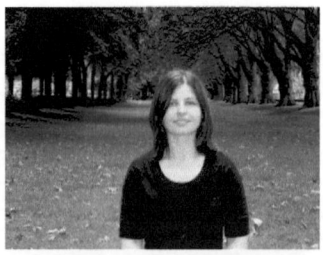

Practice 5 rounds.

Benefits:

These 3 neck exercises release tension and stiffness in the head, neck and shoulders, especially after prolonged work at the desk.

Precautions:

If you are suffering from any kind of neck related pain, injury or cervical spondylosis, please consult your doctor first before beginning any of the gentle neck exercises.

Note: *The shoulders should not move in any of the neck exercises. Please be aware while practicing neck movements that only the neck and head should move.*

Exercise 4
Shoulder Rotation

Preparation: Sit in a crossed-legged position on the floor with your back straight (*or you may sit on the chair with your back straight if you find it difficult to sit on the floor*).

Place your fingers on your shoulders with elbows down.

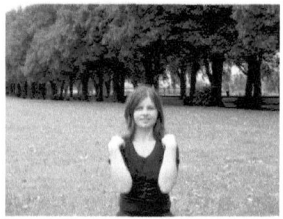 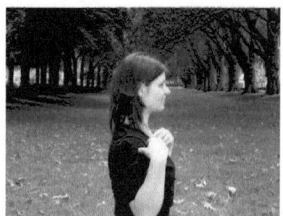

Step1: As you inhale rotate your shoulders upward (*elbows going up towards the ceiling as shown in the picture below*).

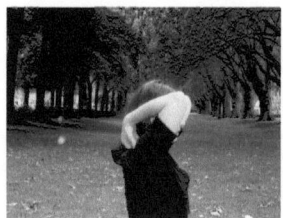

Step2: As you exhale fully rotate your shoulders downward (elbows going down towards the floor as shown in picture below).

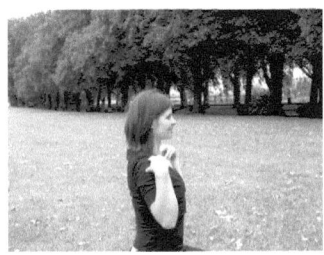

This completes one round.

Practice 5 rounds clockwise and 5 rounds anticlockwise.

Benefits:

This shoulder movement releases the strain of driving, long hours of office work and also helps in bringing mobility to tight shoulders.

Following 2 exercises are helpful in relieving tension in hands and wrists caused by prolong hours of working on computers or using your blackberry.

Exercise 5

Hand clenching

Preparation: Bring your arms straight in front of you, at the shoulder level.

Step1. As you inhale open your hands, keeping your palms down. Stretch your fingers as wide as you can.

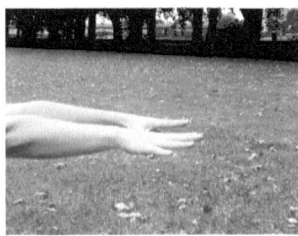

Step2. As you exhale make fists with your fingers.

This completes one round.

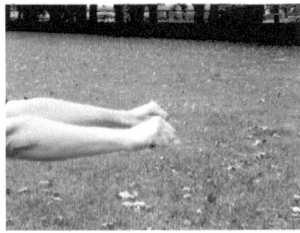

Repeat 20 times.

Exercise 6

Hand Stretch movement

Preparation: Either stand straight with feet together or sit in a cross leg position, interlocking the fingers and placing the palms on the chest as shown in picture.

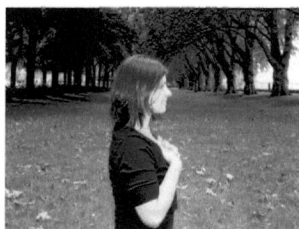

Step 1: Now inhale and stretch out the arms with palms facing outside as shown in the picture.

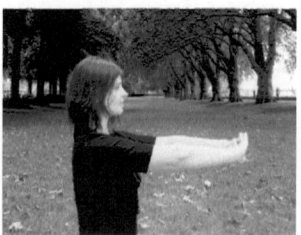

Step 2: Exhale and bring the palms back on the chest.

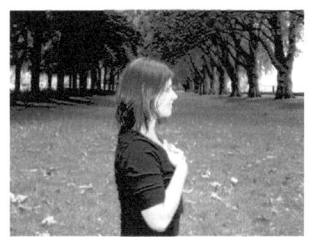

This is one round. Please practice about 5 to 10 rounds as per your comfort level. Never strain in any position.

Note: If tiredness is felt at any point during any gentle exercises, please lie down on your back on the floor for couple of minutes and practice deep breathing.

Exercise 7

Eye exercises

Eye exercises help to improve the eyesight. These exercises are very helpful if you work for long hours sitting in front of a computer.

Eye movement (a) Up and down

Preparation: Sit in a crossed-legged position on the floor with your back straight or you may sit on the chair with your back straight if you find it difficult to sit on the floor.

Step 1: Begin with your eyes in the centre position and look in front of you (Picture below).

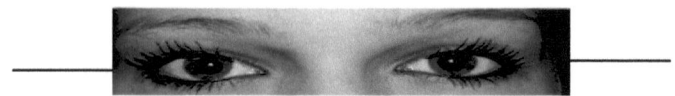

Step 2: Slowly take your eyeballs up (Picture below).

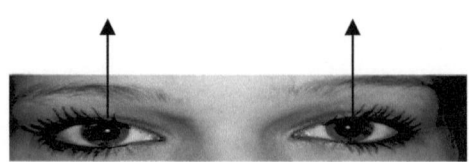

Step 3: Now slowly take your eyeballs down (Picture below).

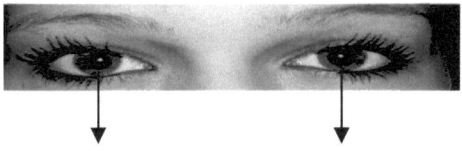

Step 4: Slowly bring your eyeballs in the centre position (Picture below).

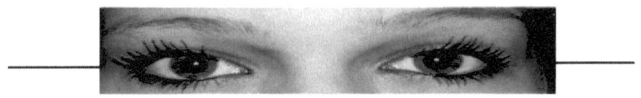

This is one round. Practice 5 rounds. After practice 5 rounds, please close your eyes gently for the next 6 breaths.

Eye exercise (b): Side to side

Step 1: Begin with your eyes in the centre position (Picture below).

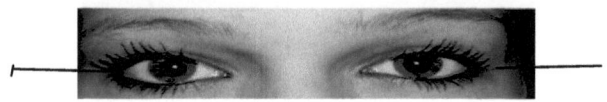

Step 2: Slowly take your eyeballs to your left side (Picture below).

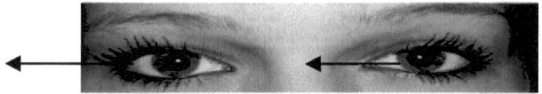

Step 3: Now slowly take your eyeballs to your right side (Picture below).

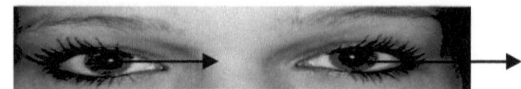

Step 4: Slowly bring your eyeballs in the centre position (Picture below).

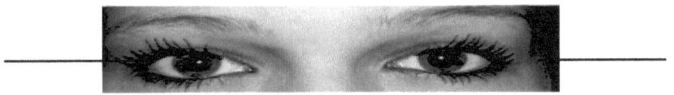

This is one round. Practice 5 rounds. After practicing 5 rounds, close your eyes gently for the next 6 breaths.

Eye exercise (c): Diagonal movement (upper left to lower right).

Step 1: Begin with your eyes in the centre position.

Step 2: Slowly take your eyeballs to your *upper* left hand corner of the wall (Picture below).

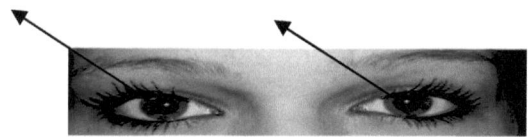

Step 3: Now slowly take your eyeballs to your *lower* right hand corner of the wall (Picture below).

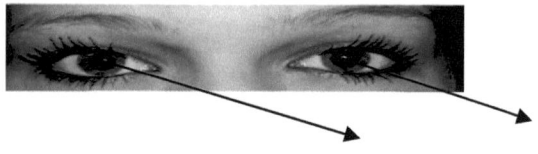

Step 4: Slowly bring your eyeballs in the centre position.

This is one round. Practice 5 rounds. After practicing 5 rounds, close your eyes gently for the next 6 breaths.

Eye exercise (d) Diagonal movement (upper right to lower left).

Step 1: Begin with your eyes in the centre position (Picture below).

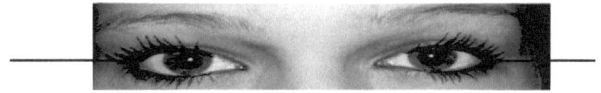

Step 2: Slowly take your eyeballs to your *upper* right hand corner of the wall (Picture below).

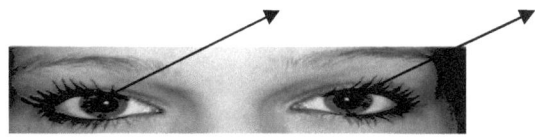

Step 3: Now slowly take your eyeballs to your *lower* left hand corner of the wall (Picture below).

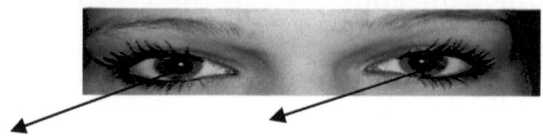

Step 4: Slowly bring your eyeballs in the centre position (Picture below).

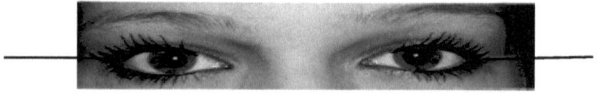

This is one round. Please practice 5 rounds. After practicing 5 rounds, please close your eyes gently for the next 6 breaths.

Note: *While doing eye exercises, please observe that you are moving your eyes only and not your head or neck.*

If you find any inconvenience during eye exercises, please stop the practice and first consult your yoga teacher or your doctor.

Exercise 8

Cat stretch

Come up in the position as shown in the picture below with your knees under your hips and your palms under your shoulders.

Your wrists, elbows and shoulders are in line and perpendicular to the floor. Centre your head in a neutral position, eyes looking at the floor (picture below).

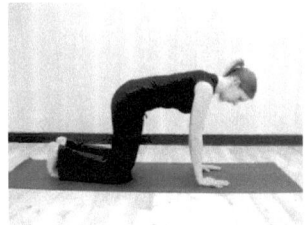

While inhaling slowly and deeply, lift your head up and bring your spine down within your comfort level as shown in the picture below.

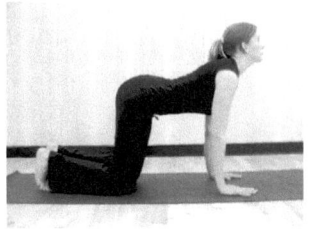

As you slowly exhale bring you head down and round your spine toward the ceiling and contract your abdomen (picture below).

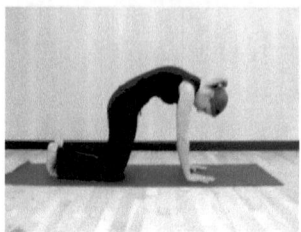

This inhalation and exhalation complete one round. You can practice 5 to 10 rounds.

This is a very good exercise for improving flexibility of the spine and it is especially helpful after long hours of sitting in the office or driving to release stiffness from the back.

Cautions

In case of neck injury and pregnancy, please practice it under guidance of an experienced yoga teacher only.

Exercise 9

Half Sun Salutation:

This concept of half sun salutation you will not find in other yoga books.

While conducting yoga sessions for various corporate organizations, I realized that full sun salutation postures are inconvenient for many people, especially those who are suffering from carpel tunnel syndrome, very weak wrists or having very stiff body, i.e. I have customized this concept of half sun salutation so that more people can do it even the one with weaker wrists and very stiff body till the time your body becomes ready for full sun salutation.

Step 1:

Stand in a straight position with your feet together and hands by your side as shown in picture below.

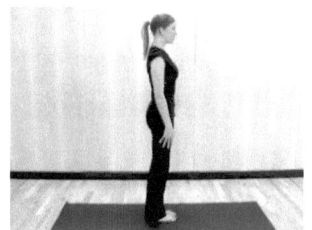

Step 2:

Inhale deeply and stretch both of your arms over the head and gently arch your back as shown in picture below. Always remember all movements of the body should be slow and without any jerks.

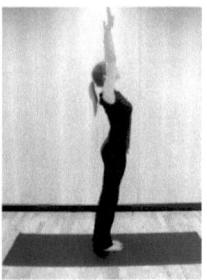

Step 3:

As you exhale bend forward, putting your hands on the floor next to your feet as shown in picture below.

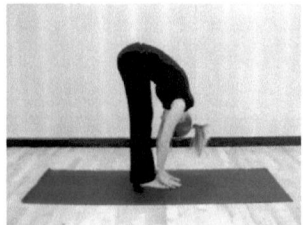

(Do not strain yourself. In case if you are having back pain, please do not bend forward fully or if you find it difficult to keep your legs straight then please slightly bend your knees as shown in picture below).

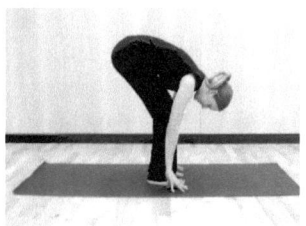

Your fingers are in line with your toes. Bring your head toward your knees.

Step 4:

While inhaling stretch your right foot back as far as possible comfortably, placing the right knee on the floor and look up as shown in picture below.

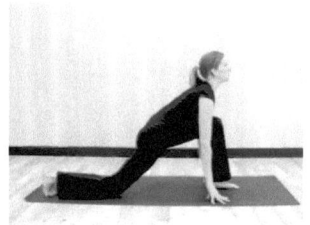

Step 5: Exhale and bring your right foot forward as shown in the picture below.

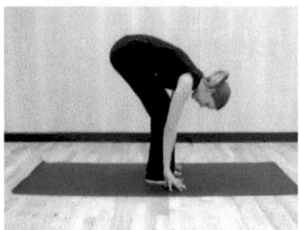

Step 6: Inhale and stretch your arms up as shown in the picture below.

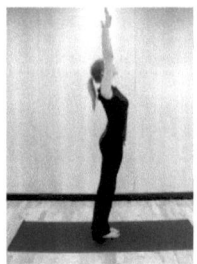

Step 7:

Exhale and bring your arms down, stand in the straight position with your feet together and hands by your side (picture below).

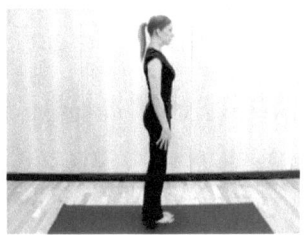

Now try the same movement with the left leg.

This completes one round.

Practice 3 to 6 rounds initially depending upon your comfort level.

Remember to combine each body movement with your breath. Breath should flow slowly, smoothly and without any jerk.

Precautions: In case of suffering from high blood pressure, hernia, pregnancy or if you had a stroke earlier, please either **avoid doing these postures** or practice it carefully **only** in presence of a qualified and experienced yoga trainer only.

Exercise 10

Full Sun Salutation:

The sun salutation is a yogic exercise for warming up the body by alternatively bending the body forward and backward. *It should be practice after gentle yoga and half sun salutation and before starting other yoga postures.*

The sun salutation exercise consists of 12 postures. The first and last postures of sun salutation are same. *The best way to learn this yogic exercise is to first become familiar with each yoga posture individually* and then practice it as a whole for some time and later on it should be synchronized with the breath.

Breathing principle: Inhale during expansion of chest (during backward bending posture) and

Exhale during compression of the chest and abdomen (during forward bending posture).

Sun salutation exercises step by step:

Posture 1:

Stand straight with your feet together and hands by your side as shown in the picture.

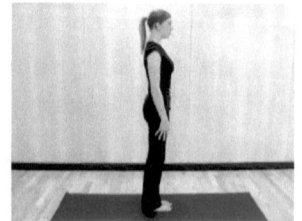

Posture 2:

Now with inhalation stretch both of your arms over the head and gently arch your back as shown in picture.

Always remember all movements of body should be slow and without any jerk.

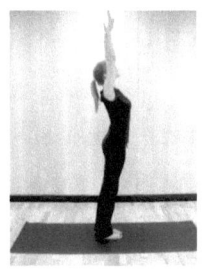

Posture 3:

As you exhale bend forward, putting your hands on the floor and your fingers are in line with your toes. Bring your head toward your knees as shown in the picture.

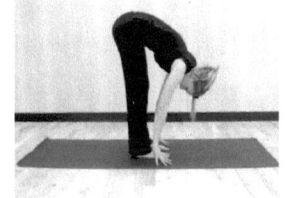

Do not strain yourself (*In case if you are having back pain, please do not bend forward fully or if you find it difficult to keep your legs straight then please slightly bend your knees as shown in the picture*).

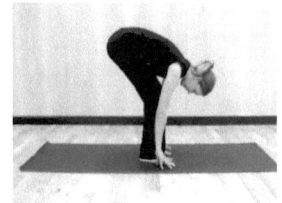

Posture 4:

While inhaling, stretch your right foot back as far as possible and place your right knee on the floor and look in front of you as shown in the picture.

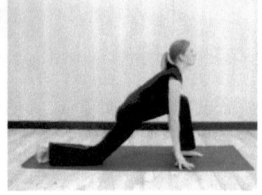

Posture 5:

Retain the breath in this pose for a moment **(fraction of a second)** while bringing the other leg back as shown in the picture.

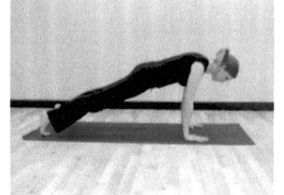

Posture 6:

While exhaling drop your knees to the floor.

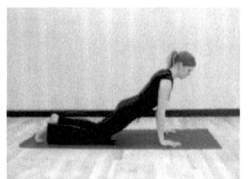

Lower your chest straight down onto the ground, between your hands. Bring your forehead (or chin) to the floor.

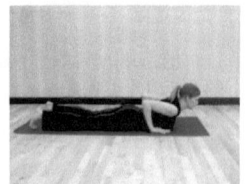

Posture 7:

While inhaling lift your head and chest up. Legs and hips remain on the ground as shown in the picture. This position is also known as cobra pose.

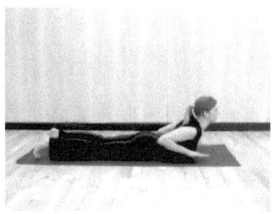

For beginners it is good if palms are above the floor.

(In some of the yoga classes by famous yoga teachers, you might find people putting too much pressure on their palms to lift their upper body up as if the body is made up of rubber and making it looks very impressive as shown in the picture below).

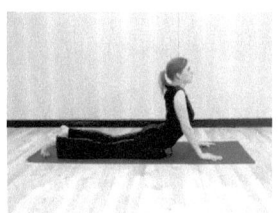

However **this posture is <u>quite harmful</u> for your body if your back is stiff and you may end up injuring your back by practicing this impressive pose.** Please be careful and **avoid** practicing this posture as <u>shown in the picture above</u>.

Posture 8:

As you exhale raise your hips up (as in inverted V pose). Your head is between your arms and very gently you can stretch the heels towards the floor within your comfort level.

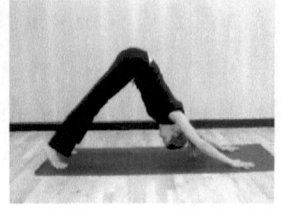

Posture 9:

While inhaling bring your right foot forward between your hands, placing your left knee on the floor. Fingers and toes are in line while looking up.

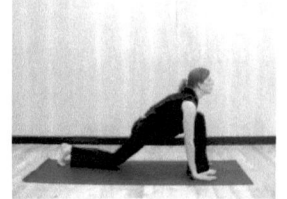

Posture 10:

While exhaling bring your left foot forward between your palms. Keep your knees straight.

(*If not comfortable bend your knees and bring your forehead towards your knees*).

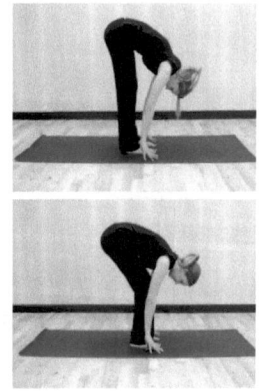

Posture 11:

As you inhale, stretch up and bring your arms straight up over your head and gently arch your back.

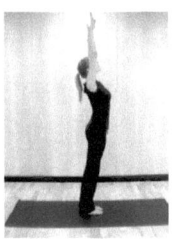

Posture 12:

While exhaling slowly drop your arms down next to your side and relax. This position is same as the starting position.

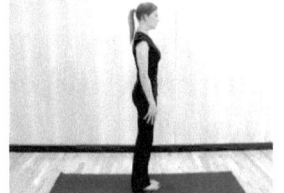

After 12 yoga postures as described above please repeat the same 12 steps with your left leg.

The combination of 12 steps with the right leg and 12 steps with left leg *complete one round.*

After completing one round take a break and observe your next 3 breaths in the standing position (posture 12).

(Please remember to take a break after every one round).

Beginners can do daily up to 6 rounds. One can increase the number of rounds to 12 after practicing at least for 8 – 12 weeks regularly.

Note: After practicing sun salutation exercise, lie down on the floor on your back and relax your whole body. Observe your breath *(please do not control the breath, only observe your breath) till the point your breath comes to normal speed.* For some people breath can come to normal speed within half a minute and for some it may take more time.

Once you notice that your breath is running at perfectly normal speed, practice slow, smooth and deep abdominal breathing for one minute before starting other yoga postures.

Benefits:

Sun salutation exercise has tremendous benefits. It helps in loosening up the joints, stretching & massaging muscles and internal organs of the body.

Its regular practice helps in improving digestion and blood circulation, reduces excess weight, removes constipation, strengthens the leg and arm muscles and makes the spine supple, etc.

Precautions: In case of suffering from carpal tunnel syndrome, severe lower back pain, high blood pressure, hernia, pregnancy or if you had a stroke earlier, **avoid doing this exercise** or practice it carefully <u>**only**</u> in presence of a qualified and experienced yoga trainer.

Exercise 11

Single Leg Raise pose

Breathing:

Inhale – while raising leg up slowly.

Exhale – while lowering leg down slowly.

Step by step method:

Preparation: Lie on your back with your palms flat on the floor and arms alongside the thighs. Keep your legs together and feet relaxed.

Step 1: As you inhale slowly raise your right leg as high as comfortably possible (max up to 90 degree) as shown in the picture.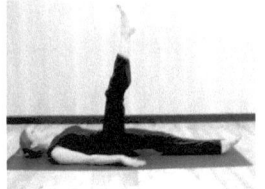

Step 2: And as you exhale lower your right leg back to the floor.

Now repeat these above 2 steps with your left leg. This completes one round.

Keep breathing throughout the practice and do 3 rounds.

Note: This is comparatively easy and safe leg-lifting exercise because it is not likely to strain a sensitive back. This posture keeps the pelvis and lower back stabilized against the floor, makes it easy and comfortable, however if you find it strenuous then please consult your yoga trainer first.

Benefits: This is a good exercise for strengthening the abdominal muscles.

Exercise 12

Single Leg Lock pose

Step by step method:

Step 1: Lie down on your back on the floor with your right knee bent towards the chest and keep your left leg relaxed and straight.

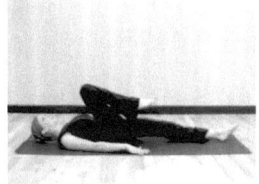

Step2: Interlock your fingers below the right knee.

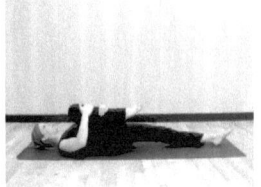

Step 3: First inhale deeply in lying position and then **while exhaling,** slowly raise your head or your chin up towards your right knee.

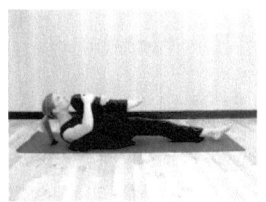

(Raise your head or chin towards your right knee to the point where you feel comfortable)

Step 4: Now while **inhaling,** slowly come down to the lying position.

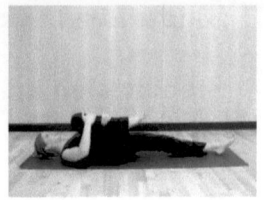

Release the right knee and repeat the same with your left leg. This will complete one round.

Practice 3 - 6 rounds.

Benefits:

It is very effective in removing unwanted wind from the body.

It is also helpful in removing constipation.

Precautions: People suffering from slipped disc or sciatica should avoid this posture or consult an experienced yoga teacher before practicing the pose.

Exercise 13

Spinal Twist

Step by step method:

Preparation: Lie flat on your back with your legs straight and palms facing down.

Step 1: Bend the right knee and place the right foot on the floor by the left knee.

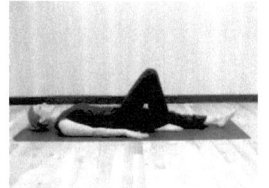

Then place your left hand on top of the right knee, as shown in picture.

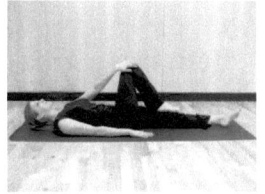

Step 2: As you exhale, bring your right knee down towards the floor on the left side of your body, turning around 45 degree left side or half way and turn your head to the right side of your body.

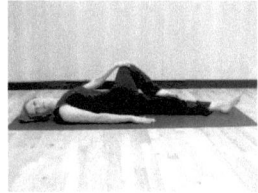

(Note: *In this position your right arm and your right shoulder should be touching the floor comfortably*).

Now hold this posture for about 30 seconds and keep breathing naturally.

Step 3: As you inhale slowly return to the centre.

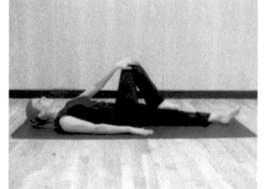

Step 4: Repeat on the other side (this completes one round).

Benefits: This yoga posture helps in releasing tightness and tiredness in the lower back and it is excellent for you, if you have a job which involves sitting on the chair for long hours.

Caution: If you experience pain at any stage, please make sure that you are not overstretching.

Exercise 14

The Dolphin

This yoga exercise strengthens the arms and shoulders.

This exercise can be done in 2 ways. If you have never done it before you can try the beginner way and after some time you can try the advanced way.

Breathing:

Inhale – while pushing the torso back

Exhale – while coming forward

Dolphin exercise For Beginners:

Step by step method:

Preparation: Place your forearms on the floor in front of you in a triangular shape with your fingers interlocked & knees on the floor as shown in the picture.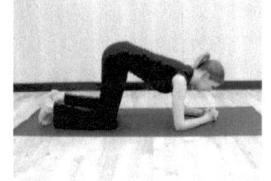

Step 1: While exhaling slowly move forward as shown in the picture.

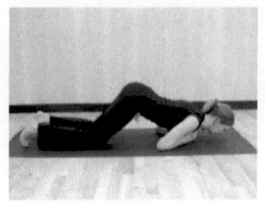

Step 2: Inhaling and come back to original position.

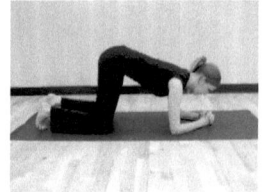

This completes one round. Practice 5 to 10 rounds.

After practicing 5 to 10 rounds relax in the Child's pose described later in this book.

Dolphin exercise for advance practitioners:

Place your forearms on the floor in front of you in a triangular shape with your fingers interlocked & straighten your legs to the V- shape position as shown in the picture.

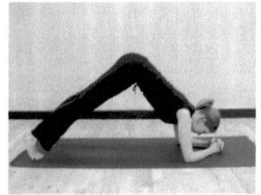

Step 1: While exhaling slowly move forward with your legs straight as shown in the picture.

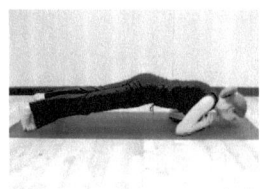

Step 2: Inhaling and come back to original position as shown in the picture.

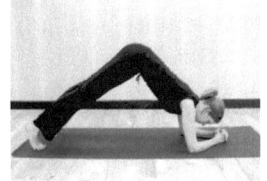

This completes one round. Practice between 5 - 10 rounds.

After practicing 5 to 10 rounds bend your knees and relax in the Child's pose described later in this book.

Benefits:

It develops upper body, abdominal and back strength.

Note:

The closer your feet are to your elbows, the more strength you will need to accomplish this movement.

Exercise 15

Shoulder stand

The Shoulder stand is an inverted yoga pose and benefits all parts of the body. This is one of the most important and beneficial yoga pose hence known as the queen of all the yoga postures.

This pose reverses the action of gravity on the body. In this posture the breath becomes slow and deep *if done correctly.*

Breathing:

Inhale – while lifting your legs up
Exhale – while lowering your legs down
Breathe slowly in the final position

Step by step method:

Lie down on the floor with legs straight and feet together.

Step 1: Inhale and lift your straight legs up to a right angle as shown in **picture** while pressing your lower back against the floor (*beginners may keep their legs slightly bend*).

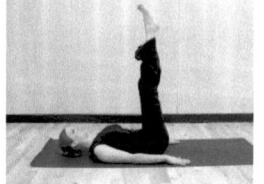

Step 2: Raise your hips off the floor and support your back with your hands and straighten your body to the point where you are comfortable and make sure that you are not straining your neck.

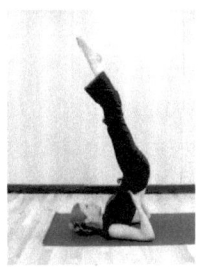

Step 3: Holding the shoulder stand posture

Please observe at this point that most of your body load is taken by your shoulders and your legs are relaxed.

While holding this posture breathe slowly and deeply. In the beginning try to hold this posture for about half a minute and slowly increase the holding time to 3 minutes.

Please remember do not hold the posture if you feel inconvenient at any time (*If you find inconvenience in your neck you can come out of posture and place a thick folded blanket under your **shoulder** and then try again*).

Coming out of the posture

Step 4: Bring your legs 45 degrees angle as shown in the picture.

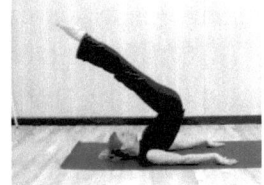

Step 5: Place your arms on the floor beside your body with palms facing down. *Then lower yourself down slowly.* The whole movement should be with control so that your body contacts the floor slowly and gently.

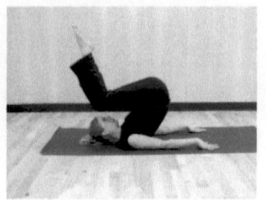

Step 6: After shoulder stand it is recommended that you relax in Savasana for about a minute.

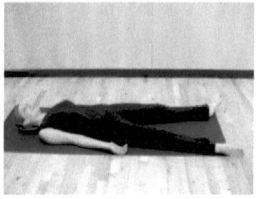

Benefits:

1. It balances the thyroid gland functions.
2. It helps participants to develop the practice of deep abdominal breathing.
3. The change in body gravity helps in bowl movement and constipation.
4. It improves the flexibility of the neck.
5. It helps in depression and insomnia.
6. Regular practice helps to prevent common cold and other nasal disturbances.

Precautions:

This yoga posture should not be practice if
(a) Suffering from neck injury,
(b) Having high blood pressure,
(c) Weak blood vessels in the eyes
(d) During Menstruation
(e) During pregnancy

Common Mistakes:

(a) Legs are tense.
(b) Turning head while in shoulder stand position.
(c) The weight is unevenly distributed, which causes the body to lean on one side
(d) Straining to bring your chin towards your chest.

(e) There is one mistake which I have observed which *most of the people make while practicing this posture including some yoga teachers as well - they put most of their body weight on their neck instead of shoulders.* Please always remember that **most** of your body weight should be on your shoulders and not on your neck.

Note:

This asana should be performed with the utmost care.

In my experience if you practice this yoga posture before sun salutation, there is possibility that you may feel backache, especially if you have stiff back. It is advisable to practice this posture after sun salutation exercise as your body would be warm up. However, if you find any pain in your back after practicing this posture then avoid this posture for the time being and practice other pose.

Exercise 16

The bridge pose

This posture helps to calm the mind and improves the digestion. It also reverses the stretch of shoulder stand.

Step 1:

Lie down on your back, bend your knees and keep your feet flat on the floor *(if you find inconvenience in your neck you may place a thick folded blanket under your shoulders)*.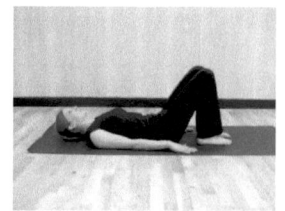

Your feet will be slightly apart. *The distance between your ankles should be about 4 -6 inches (10 to 15 centimetres).*

Step 2:

Now lift your hips up as high as possible. Hands can be supporting your back or could be on the floor with palms down as shown in the picture.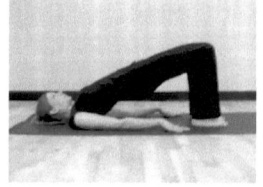

Step 3:

Hold this posture for about 30 seconds, breathe normally and then come back to the floor as shown in step 1. Initially you can begin with holding this posture for 30 seconds and later on gradually increase the holding time up to 2 minutes.

Note:

I have observed quite often in this posture that practitioner's feet and knees are turned outwards. Please make sure that your feet and knees are not turning outward and approximate distance between your ankles and knees is same.

Cautions: If you are having neck related injury, then either avoid this posture or practice it under supervision of an experienced yoga teacher only.

Exercise 17

Cobra pose

In this backbend yoga pose you lift upper part of the body away from the floor against the gravity and return to the starting position with the help of gravity.

Breathing:
Inhale – while rising up
Breathe normally while holding the pose
Exhale – while lowering down

Step by step method:

Step 1: Lie flat on the stomach with legs straight, heels and toes together. Place your hands alongside the chest, with the palms down and the elbows close to your body and rest the forehead on the floor.

Step 2: Inhale and slowly lift your forehead, neck and chest of the floor looking up. (Remember to lift your upper body up mainly using your back and neck muscles).

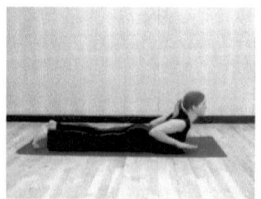

Step 3: Once you come up hold this posture and breathe normally. Please do not put much weight on your palms. Stay in this posture initially for 2 to 3 breaths.

Step 4: While exhaling gently come down.

Gradually you can increase the holding time of cobra posture up to 10 breaths as you feel more comfortable.

Benefits:

It helps to reduce backache.

It keeps the spine supple and healthy.

It helps alleviate constipation.

It stimulates the appetite.

Precautions:

People suffering from *hernia, peptic ulcer, and intestinal tuberculosis should not practice* this pose without expert guidance.

Pregnant women should not practice this yoga pose at all.

Common Mistakes:

Students use more of the arm muscles than their back muscles.

Students straighten their arms and tense their shoulders.

Note:

I have seen many times that beginners try cobra posture as shown in the picture below and also in some of the yoga classes yoga teachers are encouraging students to practice this kind of yoga position.

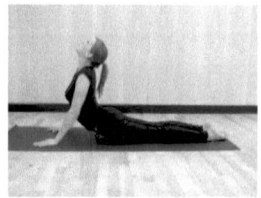

(This yoga pose is <u>not suitable</u> for <u>most</u> of the people)

This position would certainly create backache and injure those people whose back is stiff and I would strongly advise not to practice this position.

Exercise 18

Child's pose

This yoga posture stretches the spine from end to end and it is relaxing, refreshing and calming.

Breathing:

Inhale – while raising the arms above the head
Exhale – while bending forward
Breathe normally while relaxing in the pose.

Step by step method:

1.Sit on your heals, placing your palms on the thighs above the knees, keeping your spine and head straight as shown in the picture below.

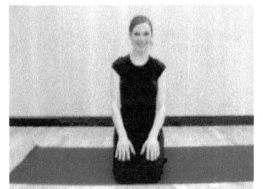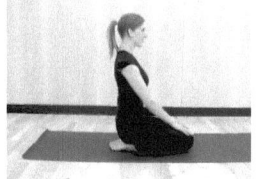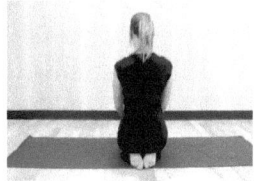

Model: Zosia Lesiecka

(If you find difficulty sitting on your heals as shown in the picture you may place small pillow under your ankles).

2. Inhale while raising your arms above the head.

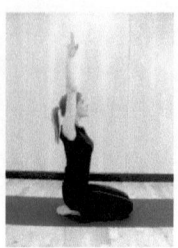

3. Bend forward while exhaling. Rest your forehead on the floor in front of your knees, and your arms alongside the legs, with the palms up.

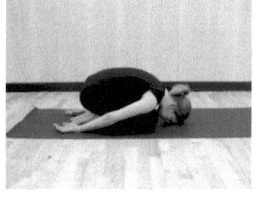

If you are a beginner, stay in this posture for about 30 seconds and later on gradually increase to 3 minutes.

Benefits:

1. It stretches the back muscles.

2. It tones the pelvic muscles.

3. It helps to relieves constipation.

Note:

If you find difficult to breathe in the child's pose then separate your knees apart.

Precautions:

This posture should not be done in case of:

(a) Pregnancy (unless modified)

(b) Diarrhoea

(c) Knee injury

(d) Vertigo

Exercise 19
Simplified Side Stretch

It is the least common movement in our ordinary day-to-day life. We twist, we bend back or forward, but we do not bend our spine to the side often. In this posture the stretch on whole side of the body takes place.

This pose is particularly useful for people who spend lots of time in sitting position. This yoga pose helps in improving the body posture.

In this side bending yoga posture, awareness should be on the breath synchronized with the body movement.

Step by step method

Step 1:
Inhale and lift your hands up as high as possible with your fingers interlocked and the palms tightly together. Now tighten all the thigh muscles and squeeze the hips together.

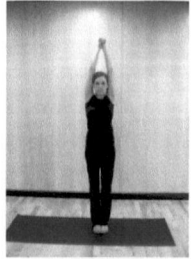

Step 2:
Exhale and bend gently to the right side within your comfort level. You will feel the stretch on your left side from your ankle to your fingertips.

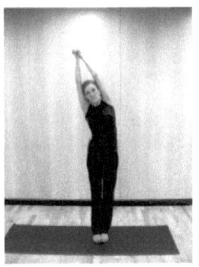

Step 3: Inhale and gently come to the centre position.

Now repeat on the other side. This would complete one round. You can practice 3 rounds.

Benefits

It improves digestion.
It helps to keep the spine flexible and healthy.

Precautions

If suffering from serious back pain, please consult an experienced yoga teacher or your doctor before beginning.
Do not overstretch yourself.
Do not twist your body

Always Remember

Relaxation pose is <u>must</u>

Exercise 20

Relaxation Pose

It is very important that after practicing yoga postures you finish your session with relaxation pose also known as Corpse pose / Savasana. This posture seems to be the easiest of all yoga posture however most difficult to master.

One needs to stay in this posture motionless with steady mind. Body can be maintained still but the difficult part is to maintain steady mind. However, with regular practice it can also be achieved and deep relaxation can be felt. This is the posture where you learn the art of conscious relaxation.

After long working hours, the natural efficiency of body and mind is decreased. Stressful moments in working life consume great amount of energy which leaves the person feeling drained.

Psychosomatic illnesses such as diabetes, hypertension, migraine, etc arise from stress which is a by product of fast pace corporate world life. If the mind is tense the stomach will also be tense and if the stomach is tense, the whole circulatory system will also be tense.

Many people wake up after sleep and they still find themselves exhausted and do not realize why?

Unless you are free from stress you can never feel relaxed but you can release the stress from your body and mind by proper relaxation exercise.

Small relaxation can be taken anytime between yoga postures whenever you feel tired, especially after sun salutation and shoulder stand.

At the end of every yoga session a complete relaxation is practiced and I recommend that everyone should also practice corpse pose before sleeping.

Relaxation Technique

Step by Step

Step 1: Lie down on the floor on your back (as shown in the picture below) in Savasana pose / Corpse pose. Arms about 15-20 cm (6 – 8 inches) away from the body and palms facing upward. Feet are slightly apart, around 30 -60 cm (1- 2 feet) and the head and spine in straight line.

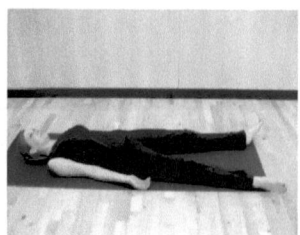

Step 2:

Now turn your neck slowly side to side 3 times.

Now take your awareness to your face muscles, tighten them and hold it for one breath and then relax them.

Now take your awareness to your arms, tighten them, make strong fists and hold it for one breath and then release them.

Take your awareness to your legs, tighten them and hold it for one breath and then release them and relax.

Now tighten the whole body, tighten … tighten and then release all your body muscles and relax.

Step 3:

After tightening and relaxing your whole body take slow and deep abdominal breaths (12 breaths). Deep breathing is very good for relaxation. (*Please note: In deep abdominal breathing abdomen rises with each inhalation and comes down with each exhalation*).

Step 4:
After 12 deep and slow abdominal breaths, observe your breath without controlling it for the next 1 minute (around 12 breaths) and then you can gently come out of the corpse pose.

Move your fingers and toes gently few times, bring your arms over the head and stretch your whole body from the tip of your fingers to the tip of your toes.

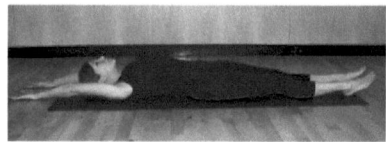

Bend your knees and turn your whole body to your left side onto the floor and stay in this position for the next 5 breaths.

Then come up in a sitting position. This completes your quick relaxation technique. If you are practicing this technique correctly you will certainly feel relaxed by now.

Benefits:
This posture calms the mind and helps in relieving stress and mild depression.
It reduces headache, fatigue and insomnia.
It helps to lower blood pressure.
It relaxes the body.

Practice Note:

Beginners in the corpse posture tend to fall asleep. Try not to move during the practice. Try not to sleep during the practice.

Precautions:

In case of back injury or *if you feel discomfort while lying on the floor with legs straight* practice this relaxation pose with your knees bent and your feet on the floor.

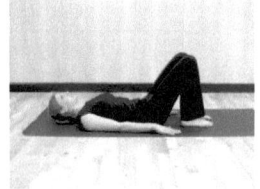

Or put some rolled towel under your knees as shown in picture.

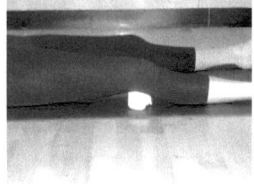

If you feel any discomfort under your neck, then you can place a thin pillow under your neck.

Wellness Monitor

Before beginning yoga exercise plan, please take couple of minutes to fill in the following wellness monitor.

	Wellness Monitor	
S.N.	Indicators	Before Beginning
1	Blood Pressure (High)	
	(Low)	
2	Lower back pain	
3	Shoulder Pain	
4	Neck Pain	
5	Finger and forearm Sprain	
6	Any Eye related issue	
7	Quality of sleep (1 to 5) (1 lowest and 5 the best, average for the week)	
8	Stress level (1 to 5) (1 lowest and 5 highest, average for the week)	
9	Overall energy level (1 to 5) (1 lowest and 5 highest)	

Yoga Practice Record

I would like to recommend that for your good health please practice yoga everyday and after the practice mark your progress in the record below.

Starting date ....

Week 1	Sun	Mon	Tue	Wed	Thu	Fri	Sat
Yoga Practice							
Week 2	Sun	Mon	Tue	Wed	Thu	Fri	Sat
Yoga Practice							
Week 3	Sun	Mon	Tue	Wed	Thu	Fri	Sat
Yoga Practice							
Week 4	Sun	Mon	Tue	Wed	Thu	Fri	Sat
Yoga Practice							

After week 4 what improvement do you feel, please write in the box below

Wellness Monitor

Now you have completed 4 week yoga practice, please take couple of minutes to fill in the following wellness monitor.

	Wellness Monitor	
S.N.	Indicators	After 4 week
1	Blood Pressure (High)	
	(Low)	
2	Lower back pain	
3	Shoulder Pain	
4	Neck Pain	
5	Finger and forearm Sprain	
6	Any Eye related issue	
7	Quality of sleep (1 to 5) (1 lowest and 5 the best, average for the week)	
8	Stress level (1 to 5) (1 lowest and 5 highest, average for the week)	
9	Overall energy level (1 to 5) (1 lowest and 5 highest)	

Yoga Practice Record

Please practice yoga everyday and after the practice mark your progress in the record below.

Practice record Week 5 to 8

Week 5	Sun	Mon	Tue	Wed	Thu	Fri	Sat
Yoga Practice							
Week 6	Sun	Mon	Tue	Wed	Thu	Fri	Sat
Yoga Practice							
Week 7	Sun	Mon	Tue	Wed	Thu	Fri	Sat
Yoga Practice							
Week 8	Sun	Mon	Tue	Wed	Thu	Fri	Sat
Yoga Practice							

After week 8 what improvement do you feel, please write in the box below

Wellness Monitor

Now you have completed 8 week of yoga practice, please take couple of minutes to fill in the following wellness monitor.

	Wellness Monitor	
S.N.	Indicators	After 8 week
1	Blood Pressure (High)	
	(Low)	
2	Lower back pain	
3	Shoulder Pain	
4	Neck Pain	
5	Finger and forearm Sprain	
6	Any Eye related issue	
7	Quality of sleep (1 to 5) (1 lowest and 5 the best, average for the week)	
8	Stress level (1 to 5) (1 lowest and 5 highest, average for the week)	
9	Overall energy level (1 to 5) (1 lowest and 5 highest)	

Yoga Practice Record

Please practice yoga everyday and after the practice mark your progress in the record below.

Practice record Week 9 to 12

Week 9	Sun	Mon	Tue	Wed	Thu	Fri	Sat
Yoga Practice							
Week 10	Sun	Mon	Tue	Wed	Thu	Fri	Sat
Yoga Practice							
Week 11	Sun	Mon	Tue	Wed	Thu	Fri	Sat
Yoga Practice							
Week 12	Sun	Mon	Tue	Wed	Thu	Fri	Sat
Yoga Practice							

After week 12 what improvement do you feel, please write in the box below

Wellness Monitor

Well done, now you have completed 12 week of yoga practice, please take couple of minutes to fill in the following wellness monitor.

	Wellness Monitor	
S.N.	Indicators	After 12 week
1	Blood Pressure (High)	
	(Low)	
2	Lower back pain	
3	Shoulder Pain	
4	Neck Pain	
5	Finger and forearm Sprain	
6	Any Eye related issue	
7	Quality of sleep (1 to 5) (1 lowest and 5 the best, average for the week)	
8	Stress level (1 to 5) (1 lowest and 5 highest, average for the week)	
9	Overall energy level (1 to 5) (1 lowest and 5 highest)	

Dear Yoga Practitioner,

While practicing yoga exercises if you come across any question, you are welcome to send us your query at: info@subodhgupta.com

More information about us is available at

www.subodhgupta.com

You are also welcome to send us your experience about yoga if you would like them to be published on our website.

I wish you good health and happiness in your life.

With Best Regards
Subodh Gupta

Workshops and Yoga classes at workplace in London

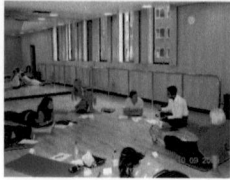 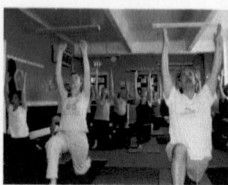 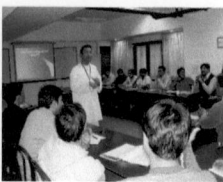

We provide following workshops and yoga classes for corporate organizations and Celebrities in London.

(1) Regular Yoga Classes at work place for Managing Stresses.

(2) Half hour/ One hour Yoga Workshops for rejuvenation during day long Conferences and board meetings.

(3) 4 hours workshop on work life balance / Stress Management.

(4) 6 week weight management program for celebrities

For more details please contact:

Barbara Tomasik
Indian Foundation for Scientific Yoga and Stress Management
44(0)7966275913 (London)
info@subodhgupta.com, barbara@subodhgupta.com

www.subodhgupta.com

Our other Published books:

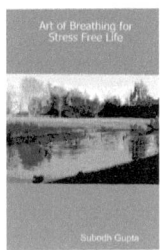

Art of Breathing
for
Stress free Life

The Only book on human breathing techniques for managing stress with clearly illustrated photographs and practical instructions. This book is ideal for busy people who lead a hectic life style.

ISBN 978-1-84799-047-1

Library of Congress Control Number: 2007907962
Soft cover /£9.95/ 56 pages

"Valuable & to the point breathing techniques to reduce stress in short time. This book is must for the corporate world."
---Yogesh Garg, Chairman, Infraline Energy Research and Information Services

For more details please visit our website:
www.subodhgupta.com/books.html

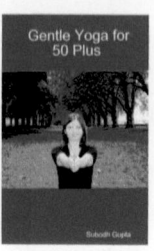

Gentle Yoga for 50 Plus

"A perfect gift of health for your parents"

The only book on Gentle Yoga for people in the age group of 50 plus.

This book is specifically for those people who feel their body is stiff or have never done yoga before and want to start yoga practice in the safest possible way to achieve healthy body and mind.

The exercises explained in this book are also beneficial if suffering from arthritis or rheumatism.

"Those who have associate the term "yoga" with words like "difficult," "time-consuming," "boring," or "painful," will find **Gentle Yoga for 50 Plus** *a light hearted, encouraging, and easy-to-follow introduction to a practice which has long been known to provide a multitude of benefits for its practitioners."*

- **ForeWord Clarion Reviews**

ISBN 978-1-84799-149-2

Library of Congress Control Number: 2007908785
Soft cover/ £9.95/ 56 pages

For more details please visit our website:
www.subodhgupta.com/books.html

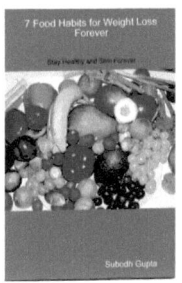

7 Food Habits for Weight Loss *Forever*

Stay Healthy and Slim *Forever*

"For anybody who wants to lose weight and gain health forever"

"Managing perfect body weight is not a complicated rocket science. Our body is made up of food which we eat during our day to day life. If we are overweight or obese at the moment then one thing is certain that the food which we eat is not good."

Healthy Food Habits = Good Health + Perfect Body weight *forever*

ISBN 978-0-9556882-0-1
Page 68 / Soft Cover / £9.95

For more details please visit our website:
www.subodhgupta.com/books.html

All our books are also available at Amazon.co.uk

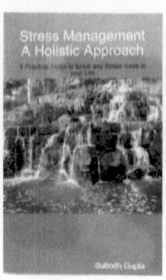

Stress Management A Holistic Approach
5 Practical Steps to solve any Stress issue in your life

"For anyone who wants to live a Stress free life"

Many illnesses such as diabetes, migraine, asthma, ulcer and even cancer arise because of excessive Stress over the period of time.

This book presents a holistic and practical approach for Managing Stress. If there is a problem then there has to be a solution and this book is all about solution.

You may have any kind of problem or issue in your life, once you follow the 5 steps described in this book you are on your way to Stress free life.

ISBN 978-0-9556882-1-8

Page 80 / Soft Cover / £7.95

For more details please visit our website:
www.subodhgupta.com/books.html

All our books are also available at Amazon.co.uk

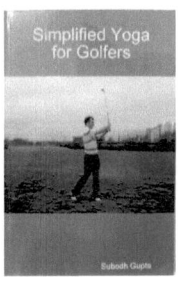

Simplified Yoga for Golfers

The yoga plan in this book is carefully designed for people who play golf.

A strong and flexible body creates the foundation for a injury-free golf game. Simplified Yoga poses described in this book will not only strengthen the muscles but will also help to bring flexibility.

All the yoga poses described in this book are translated in English name.

Flexibility + Strength = Injury free Golf Game

ISBN 978-0-9556882-3-2
Page 96 / Soft Cover / £24.95

For more details please visit our website:
www.subodhgupta.com/books.html

All our books are also available at Amazon.co.uk, Barnes and Nobles.

Notes

Notes

www.ingramcontent.com/pod-product-compliance
Ingram Content Group UK Ltd.
Pitfield, Milton Keynes, MK11 3LW, UK
UKHW041435180426
11947UKWH00007B/450